Ice Baths

Beginners Guide

Boost Recovery, Improve Performance, & Enhance Wellness

© *Copyright 2021 - All rights reserved.*

The content contained within this book may not be reproduced, duplicated, or transmitted without direct written permission from the author or the publisher.

Under no circumstances will any blame or legal responsibility be held against the publisher, or author, for any damages, reparation, or monetary loss due to the information contained within this book. Either directly or indirectly. You are responsible for your own choices, actions, and results.

Legal Notice:

This book is copyright protected. This book is only for personal use. You cannot amend, distribute, sell, use, quote or paraphrase any part, or the content within this book, without the consent of the author or publisher.

Disclaimer Notice:

Please note the information contained within this document is for educational and entertainment purposes only. All effort has been executed to present accurate-to-date, reliable, complete information. No warranties of any kind are declared or implied. Readers acknowledge that the author is not engaging in the rendering of legal, financial, medical, or professional advice. The content within this book has been derived from various sources. Please consult a licensed professional before attempting any techniques outlined in this book.

By reading this document, the reader agrees that under no circumstances is the author responsible for any losses, direct or indirect, which are incurred as a result of the use of the information contained within this document, including, but not limited to, — errors, omissions, or inaccuracies

Contents

Introduction 7

What is an ice bath? 9

The Origin of Ice Baths 11

Benefits of taking ice baths 12

Preparing for your first ice bath 15

Setting up your ice bath 18

How long to stay in an ice bath 20

Techniques for managing discomfort 22

Getting the most out of your ice bath 24

Post-ice bath recovery and care 26

Safety considerations for ice baths 28

Incorporating ice baths into your routine 30

Alternatives to full-body ice baths 32

Common misconceptions about ice baths 34

Frequently asked questions about ice baths 36

Testimonials and success stories 38

Famous Ice Bathers 40

In Conclusion **42**

Introduction

Welcome to "Ice Baths, Beginners Guide: How to Boost Recovery, Improve Performance, and Enhance Wellness."

Whether you're an athlete looking to improve your performance or someone looking for a natural way to manage pain and inflammation, ice baths can be a powerful tool in your recovery and wellness routine.

This comprehensive guide is designed to provide you with all the information you need to get started with ice baths, including preparation, techniques, safety considerations, and alternative forms of cold therapy.

We'll also address common misconceptions and frequently asked questions to help you make informed decisions about incorporating ice baths into your routine.

With testimonials and success stories from individuals who have already experienced the benefits of ice baths, we hope to inspire and empower you to take your recovery and wellness to the next level.

Let's dive in!

What is an ice bath?

An ice bath is a form of cold water therapy where the body is immersed in cold water, typically with ice added, for a short period of time. It's a popular practice among athletes, particularly in endurance sports, as it's believed to help reduce muscle soreness, and inflammation, and can also promote faster recovery after intense workouts or competitions.

Ice baths can be taken in a bathtub, or a large container filled with cold water and ice, and the temperature of the water is usually between 50 to 59 degrees Fahrenheit (10 to 15 degrees Celsius). The recommended duration of an ice bath varies but typically should last anywhere from 5 to 20 minutes depending on individual tolerance and experience.

While ice baths can offer several benefits, they can also be uncomfortable and can be risky, especially if you have certain medical conditions or if you are pregnant. If you do have any medical conditions, it's recommended that you consult a healthcare professional before trying them, to determine whether they are safe for you.

Following proper safety protocols to prevent hypothermia or other adverse effects is important.

The Origin of Ice Baths

Ice bath therapy, also known as cold water immersion therapy, has been used for centuries in various cultures for its therapeutic benefits. The ancient Greeks and Romans, for example, used cold water immersion as a form of therapy for various ailments and injuries.

In modern times, the use of ice bath therapy became popular in the early 20th century, particularly among athletes and sports teams. It was initially used to help reduce swelling and inflammation after injuries, as well as to relieve muscle soreness and speed up recovery time.

Over time, the benefits of ice bath therapy have been further studied and documented, and it has become a widely used practice in various fields, including sports medicine, physical therapy, mental health therapy and even the beauty industry.

Benefits of taking ice baths

Ice baths can have many benefits for both physical and mental health, they can help reduce muscle soreness and inflammation that can occur after intense exercise, as the cold water is believed to constrict blood vessels, which can help reduce muscle swelling and inflammation. By reducing inflammation and promoting blood flow, ice baths can help speed up recovery time after exercise, allowing athletes to train more frequently and with greater intensity.

Exposure to cold water stimulates blood circulation and increases oxygen flow to the body's tissues and organs. When the body is exposed to cold water, blood vessels near the skin's surface constrict, which helps conserve heat and maintain core body temperature. At the same time, the body's natural response is to increase heart rate and blood pressure, which can help to increase blood flow and oxygen delivery to the body's tissues and organs.

Additionally, exposure to cold water can activate the sympathetic nervous system, which is responsible for the "fight or flight" response. This can lead to the release of adrenaline and other hormones, which can increase heart rate and blood pressure, further promoting blood flow and oxygen delivery to the body's tissues.

Prolonged exposure to cold water can lead to hypothermia, which is a dangerous condition where the body's core temperature drops too low. It's important to always take appropriate safety precautions when engaging in activities that involve exposure to cold water.

Some people find that taking ice baths can help reduce stress and promote a sense of calmness and mental clarity. Cold water can trigger the body's "fight or flight" response, which releases hormones like adrenaline and cortisol which can help to reduce stress and anxiety. Additionally, the experience of taking an ice bath can be mentally challenging, and some people find that the sense of accomplishment after completing the bath can contribute to a sense of calmness and mental ease.

There is also some evidence to suggest that exposure to cold water can stimulate the immune system and help the body fight off infections and illnesses, although research in this area is still limited. Some studies have found that exposure to cold water can increase the production of certain immune cells and cytokines, which are molecules that help to regulate the immune response. It has also been shown to increase the activity of natural killer cells, which are a type of white blood cell that plays an important role in the body's defense against viruses and cancer cells.

Moreover, cold water exposure has been used in various traditional practices, such as hydrotherapy, to support the immune system and promote healing. However, more research is needed to fully understand the mechanisms behind cold water exposure's immune-boosting effects and determine its effectiveness in preventing or treating infections and illnesses.

It's important to note that while cold water exposure may have potential health benefits, it should always be approached with caution and under appropriate supervision, as prolonged exposure to cold water can be dangerous and lead to hypothermia or other health complications.

Preparing for your first ice bath

If you have never had an ice bath before, try something to ease yourself in and climatise your body.

Cold showers can be a good way to start incorporating cold water exposure into your routine. Cold showers can be invigorating and energising and can provide some of the benefits of cold water exposure without the risks associated with more intense forms of exposure, such as ice baths.

Starting with shorter cold showers and gradually increasing the duration and intensity of the exposure can help your body adjust to the colder temperatures and minimise the risk of hypothermia or other adverse effects. It's also important to listen to your body and stop the cold shower if you feel uncomfortable or experience any negative symptoms.

In terms of potential benefits, some people report that cold showers can help to increase alertness and focus, reduce muscle soreness and inflammation, improve skin and hair health, and even boost the immune system. However, it's important to keep in mind that more research is needed to confirm these findings.

Overall, if you're interested in trying cold water exposure, starting with shorter cold showers and gradually increasing the duration and intensity of the exposure can be a good way to get started while minimising the risks.

If you're planning to try an ice bath for the first time, here are some more steps to help you prepare:

Ice baths can be taken in a bathtub or a large container, but make sure the container is sturdy and can hold enough water to submerge your body.

You will need a container, ice, a thermometer to measure the water temperature, a timer, and towels.

Fill the container with cold water and add ice until the temperature reaches between 50 to 59 degrees Fahrenheit (10 to 15 degrees Celsius). Use the thermometer to ensure the temperature is accurate.

Wear comfortable clothing that allows for easy movement and quick drying after the ice bath. Swimsuits or workout clothes are good options.

Ice baths can be uncomfortable, especially for beginners. Take some deep breaths and mentally prepare yourself before getting into the water.

Breathing exercises can be a useful tool for mental preparation and can help to promote calmness and focus. There are many different breathing techniques that can be used for mental preparation, but one of the most popular is called "box breathing."

Box breathing involves inhaling for a count of four, holding the breath for a count of four, exhaling for a count of four, and then holding the breath for a count of four before beginning the cycle again. The goal is to maintain a steady and even breath throughout the exercise, with an emphasis on the exhale to help promote relaxation and calmness.

Other breathing exercises that can be useful for mental preparation include deep breathing, alternate nostril breathing, and rhythmic breathing. These exercises can help to slow down the breathing rate, reduce stress and anxiety, and promote a sense of relaxation and mental clarity.

It's worth noting that while breathing exercises can be helpful for mental preparation, they should not be used as a substitute for professional mental health treatment if needed. If you're experiencing persistent or severe mental health symptoms, it's important to seek the guidance of a healthcare provider.

For your first ice bath, start with a short duration of 1 to 2 minutes and gradually increase the duration in subsequent sessions as your body adapts.

After the ice bath, have a warm drink ready to help raise your body temperature and promote recovery. Remember to take it slow and listen to your body. If you experience any discomfort or pain, exit the ice bath immediately.

Setting up your ice bath

Choose a location that is spacious enough to accommodate the container for your ice bath. It should also be an area that can get wet, such as a bathroom or outdoor area.

Choose a container that is large enough to submerge your body comfortably, and sturdy enough to hold the weight of the water and ice. A plastic storage bin or a large cooler are good options.

Fill the container with cold water. Use a thermometer to measure the temperature of the water and adjust accordingly to reach a temperature between 50 to 59 degrees Fahrenheit (10 to 15 degrees Celsius).

Add enough ice to the water to bring the temperature down to the desired range, depending on the size of the container and the amount of ice, this may take some time.

Use a large spoon or stirrer to mix the ice and water together to ensure the temperature is consistent throughout the bath.

Use a thermometer to test the temperature of the water and adjust accordingly.

Set a timer for the desired duration of your ice bath. For beginners, start with a shorter duration of 1 to 2 minutes and gradually increase in subsequent sessions.

Have towels and warm clothing ready to dry off and warm up after the ice bath.

Remember to always use caution and take safety precautions when setting up your ice bath. Use a sturdy container, monitor the temperature of the water, and have someone nearby in case of emergency.

Don't forget your hot drink!

How long to stay in an ice bath

As mentioned previously, the recommended duration for an ice bath can vary depending on individual tolerance and experience.

For beginners, it is generally recommended to start with a shorter duration of 1 to 2 minutes and gradually increase the duration in subsequent sessions as the body adapts.

The optimal duration of an ice bath may also depend on the type and intensity of the activity being performed. For example, athletes who have just completed an intense workout or competition may benefit from a longer ice bath duration of up to 15 minutes to help reduce muscle soreness and promote recovery.

It's important to listen to your body and avoid staying in the ice bath for too long. Signs that it's time to exit the ice bath include shivering, numbness, or discomfort.

It's also important to warm up slowly after the ice bath, as sudden exposure to warm temperatures can be uncomfortable or even harmful.

Techniques for managing discomfort

Taking an ice bath can be uncomfortable, especially for beginners. Here are some techniques that can help you manage discomfort:

Focus on breathing, take deep, slow breaths to help relax your body and manage the discomfort.

Bring a book, listen to music, or watch a video to help take your mind off the discomfort.

Gradually expose your body to the cold water, starting with your feet and working your way up to your torso. This can help your body adjust to the cold temperature more easily.

Move your arms and legs to help circulate blood and warm up your body.

Mentally prepare yourself before getting into the ice bath by visualising a calming scene or repeating a mantra to help you stay focused.

Wearing a hat or warm clothing during the ice bath can help keep your head and body warm and reduce discomfort.

After the ice bath, take a warm shower or wrap yourself in warm towels to help raise your body temperature and promote recovery.

Remember that it's important to listen to your body and exit the ice bath if you experience any discomfort or pain.

Gradually increasing the duration and frequency of ice baths can help your body adapt to the cold temperature over time.

Getting the most out of your ice bath

Take an ice bath as soon as possible after an intense workout or competition. This can help reduce inflammation and muscle soreness.

Start with a shorter duration of 1 to 2 minutes and gradually increase in subsequent sessions. For athletes, a longer duration of up to 15 minutes may be beneficial.

Aim for a water temperature between 50 to 59 degrees Fahrenheit (10 to 15 degrees Celsius) to achieve the desired therapeutic effects.

Move your arms and legs to help circulate blood and promote recovery.

Consider alternating between hot and cold therapy for an even greater therapeutic effect. After the ice bath, take a warm shower or use a hot tub to help increase blood flow and promote recovery.

Drink plenty of water before and after the ice bath to help rehydrate your body.

Consider using other recovery aids, such as foam rolling or massage, to further promote recovery.

For the best results, incorporate ice baths into your regular routine, gradually increasing the frequency and duration over time as your body adapts to the cold temperature.
Remember to always listen to your body and exit the ice bath if you experience any discomfort or pain.

If you have any underlying medical conditions, it's important to consult with your healthcare provider before starting any new therapy or exercise regimen.

Post-ice bath recovery and care

After taking an ice bath, taking care of your body is important to promote recovery and avoid any potential injuries. Here are some tips for post-ice bath recovery and care:

Avoid sudden exposure to warm temperatures after an ice bath. Instead, warm up gradually by wrapping yourself in warm towels or taking a warm shower.

Drink plenty of water to help rehydrate your body and replenish any fluids lost during the ice bath.

Do some light stretching or movement exercises to help promote blood flow and prevent muscle stiffness.

Consider using other recovery aids, such as foam rolling or massage, to further promote recovery.

Allow your body to rest and recover after an ice bath. Avoid any intense exercise or activity immediately after an ice bath.

Keep an eye out for any adverse reactions, such as skin discoloration or numbness, and seek medical attention if necessary.

Gradually increase the frequency and duration of ice baths over time as your body adapts to the cold temperature.

Remember to always listen to your body and adjust your routine accordingly.

Safety considerations for ice baths

Ice baths can provide many benefits but can also be risky if not done safely. Here are some safety considerations to keep in mind when taking an ice bath:

Do not stay in the ice bath for too long as this can increase the risk of hypothermia, frostbite, and other cold-related injuries. The recommended duration for an ice bath is usually between 1 to 15 minutes, depending on individual tolerance and experience.

Gradually increase the duration and frequency of ice baths over time as your body adapts to the cold temperature. Do not attempt to take longer or more frequent ice baths than recommended.

Use a thermometer to ensure the water temperature is between 50 to 59 degrees Fahrenheit (10 to 15 degrees Celsius). Water that is too cold can increase the risk of cold-related injuries.

Drink plenty of water before and after the ice bath to avoid dehydration.

Do not take an ice bath if you have any underlying medical conditions that may be worsened by extreme cold exposure, such as Raynaud's disease or asthma.

Keep an eye out for any adverse reactions, such as skin discoloration or numbness, and seek medical attention if necessary.

Pregnant women and children should avoid taking ice baths as they may be more susceptible to cold-related injuries.

If you have any underlying medical conditions, it's important to consult with your healthcare provider before starting any new therapy or exercise regimen.

Remember to always listen to your body and adjust your routine accordingly. If you experience any discomfort or pain during an ice bath, exit the ice bath immediately.

Incorporating ice baths into your routine

If you're interested in incorporating ice baths into your routine, here are some tips to get started:

Start with shorter sessions and gradually build up to longer ones. Begin with 1 to 2 minute sessions and increase the time as your body adjusts to the cold temperature.

Incorporate ice baths into your regular routine for best results. Aim for one to three sessions per week.

Take an ice bath as soon as possible after an intense workout or competition. This can help reduce inflammation and muscle soreness.

Set up your ice bath in advance and have everything you need nearby, such as a towel and warm clothing.

Pay attention to how your body reacts to the cold temperature and adjust accordingly.

If you experience any discomfort or pain during an ice bath, exit the ice bath immediately.

Alternating between hot and cold therapy can provide additional benefits. After the ice bath, take a warm shower or use a hot tub to help increase blood flow and promote recovery.

Drink plenty of water before and after the ice bath to help rehydrate your body.

Remember to be patient and consistent with your ice bath routine. Gradually increase the duration and frequency over time as your body adapts to the cold temperature.

Alternatives to full-body ice baths

If a full-body ice bath is not for you, there are alternative ways to experience the benefits of cold therapy:

Localised cold therapy: Apply ice packs or a cold compress to a specific area of your body to reduce inflammation and promote healing.

Cold showers: Taking a cold shower for a few minutes can also help promote recovery and reduce muscle soreness.

Cryotherapy: This involves using a special chamber that exposes the body to extremely cold air for a short period of time. This can be a more controlled and targeted form of cold therapy.

Ice massage: Using a frozen water bottle or ice pack, massage a specific area of the body for several minutes to promote recovery and reduce inflammation.

Cold-water immersion: Instead of a full-body ice bath, you can immerse your legs or feet in cold water to experience some of the benefits of cold therapy.

Cooling vests: Wearing a cooling vest or other cooling garments during or after exercise can help reduce core body temperature and promote recovery.

Common misconceptions about ice baths

There are a few common misconceptions about ice baths that should be cleared up:

Ice baths are not a cure-all.

While ice baths can provide many benefits, they are not a cure-all for all injuries or conditions. Ice baths should be used as part of a comprehensive recovery plan that includes rest, proper nutrition, and other therapies.

Longer does not mean better.

There is a misconception that longer ice bath sessions provide better results. However, staying in an ice bath for too long can increase the risk of hypothermia and other cold-related injuries. The recommended duration for an ice bath is usually between 1 to 15 minutes, depending on individual tolerance and experience.

Not everyone should use ice baths.

Ice baths are not suitable for everyone, especially those with certain medical conditions or who are pregnant. It's important to consult with your healthcare provider before starting any new therapy or exercise regimen.

Ice baths are the only form of cold therapy:

While ice baths are a popular form of cold therapy, there are other ways to experience the benefits of cold therapy, such as localised cold therapy, cold showers, and cryotherapy.

Ice baths can replace proper recovery techniques:

Ice baths should be used in conjunction with other recovery techniques, such as stretching, foam rolling, and rest. Ice baths alone cannot replace proper recovery techniques.

Frequently asked questions about ice baths

Are ice baths safe?

Yes, ice baths are generally safe when done correctly and for a reasonable amount of time. However, it's important to follow proper safety protocols, such as monitoring the temperature and duration of the ice bath and having a friend or family member present.

How often should I take an ice bath?

The frequency of ice baths depends on individual preferences and needs. Most people take ice baths 1-3 times per week.

How long should I stay in an ice bath?

The recommended duration for an ice bath is usually between 1 to 15 minutes, depending on individual tolerance and experience.

How cold should the water be for an ice bath?

The water temperature should be between 50 to 60 degrees Fahrenheit (10 to 15 degrees Celsius) for an ice bath.

Can I take an ice bath if I'm pregnant?

It's not recommended for pregnant women to take ice baths or use cold therapy due to the risk of hypothermia and other complications. Consult with your healthcare provider before using any new therapies.

Can ice baths help with muscle soreness?

Yes, ice baths can help reduce muscle soreness and promote recovery after intense exercise.

What are the benefits of ice baths?

Some benefits of ice baths include reducing inflammation, promoting recovery, reducing muscle soreness, and increasing circulation.

Are there any alternatives to ice baths?

Yes, there are alternative forms of cold therapy, such as localised cold therapy, cold showers, cryotherapy, and cooling vests.

Testimonials and success stories

Here are some testimonials and success stories from individuals who have incorporated ice baths into their routines. These testimonials and success stories demonstrate the potential benefits of incorporating ice baths into a recovery and wellness routine.

John

"I've been taking ice baths after intense workouts for the past few months, and I've noticed a significant reduction in muscle soreness and inflammation. It's been a game-changer for my recovery."

Sarah

"I was skeptical about ice baths at first, but after trying it out for a few weeks, I've noticed a significant improvement in my athletic performance. I feel stronger and more energised during workouts."

Steven

"As someone who suffers from chronic back pain and inflammation, ice baths have been my lifesaver. It's one of the few things that can provide me with immediate relief and helps me manage my symptoms."

Katy

"I used to struggle with insomnia, but after incorporating ice baths into my night-time routine, I've noticed a significant improvement in the quality of my sleep. I wake up feeling more rested and rejuvenated."

Kieran

"I enjoy running marathons, and I used to dread the soreness that comes with the training, but ice baths have made a huge difference. Not only do I feel less sore, but I also feel more mentally ready for my next workout."

These testimonials and success stories demonstrate the potential benefits of incorporating ice baths into a recovery and wellness routine.

Famous Ice Bathers

There are many athletes and celebrities who have spoken publicly about their use of ice baths as part of their training or wellness routines. Here are a few examples:

LeBron James

The basketball superstar is known for his dedication to fitness and recovery and has said that he takes ice baths to help reduce inflammation and soreness after games and workouts.

Tony Robbins

The motivational speaker and life coach is a proponent of cold-water exposure, including ice baths, as a way to promote mental and physical resilience.

Laird Hamilton

The big wave surfer is a well-known advocate of cold-water therapy and has even designed his own line of ice baths called the XPT Life Pool.

Wim Hof

The Dutch extreme athlete, also known as "The Iceman," has gained notoriety for his ability to withstand extremely cold temperatures and his promotion of a method he calls the "Wim Hof Method," which includes cold exposure as one of its components.

Tom Brady

The NFL quarterback has spoken about his use of ice baths as part of his recovery routine and has even designed his own line of recovery pajamas called "TB12 Recovery Sleepwear."

While many famous people and athletes use ice baths, it's important to approach cold water exposure with caution and to seek the guidance of a healthcare professional before trying it yourself, especially if you have any underlying health conditions.

In Conclusion

In conclusion, incorporating ice baths into your recovery and wellness routine can provide numerous benefits, including improved circulation, reduced muscle soreness and inflammation, enhanced performance, and even a positive impact on mental health. However, it's important to prepare properly, manage discomfort, and prioritise safety when incorporating ice baths into your routine.

To prepare for your first ice bath, make sure you have the proper equipment and a safe and comfortable space to take your ice bath. Start with shorter durations and gradually increase the time you spend in the bath to avoid shock to your body. Techniques such as deep breathing and visualisation can help manage discomfort during your ice bath.

It's important to prioritise safety when incorporating ice baths into your routine. Never take an ice bath if you have an underlying medical condition or are pregnant, and always listen to your body and adjust your routine accordingly.

Alternatives to full-body ice baths, such as localised cold therapy and cryotherapy, can be effective options for those who cannot tolerate a full-body ice bath.

Remember, the benefits of ice baths are not limited to athletes. Anyone can benefit from incorporating ice baths into their recovery and wellness routine. With proper preparation and safety considerations, ice baths can be a powerful tool for managing pain and inflammation, improving circulation, enhancing performance, and promoting overall wellness.

We hope that this comprehensive guide has provided you with the information you need to get started with ice baths and that you feel inspired to explore this powerful tool for recovery and wellness.

Whether you're an athlete looking to improve your performance or someone looking for a natural way to manage pain and inflammation, ice baths can be a powerful addition to your routine.

Thank you for reading, I hope you enjoyed this simple guide and I hope you enjoy your new ice bath experience.

Stay safe, stay cool, and have fun!

Printed in Great Britain
by Amazon